Neoantigen Cancer Vaccine

The Cancer Vaccine Revolution and the

New Era of Cancer Treatment

Dr. Quinn M. Rios

Table of Content

INTRODUCTION

CHAPTER 1

WHAT IS CANCER?
RISK FACTORS FOR CANCER
CANCER PREVENTION
TYPES OF CANCER
GENERAL SIGNS AND SYMPTOMS OF CANCER
IMPORTANCE OF DETECTING CANCER EARLIER
CANCER TREATMENTS

CHAPTER 2

CANCER VACCINE
TYPES OF CANCER VACCINES
THE EVOLUTION OF CANCER VACCINES
THE EMERGENCE OF NEOANTIGENS
THE NEOANTIGEN REVOLUTION IN CANCER VACCINES
FUTURE OF CANCER VACCINES

CHAPTER 3

THE SCIENCE BEHIND NEOANTIGENS

WHAT ARE NEOANTIGENS?

HOW ARE NEOANTIGENS GENERATED?

HOW DOES THE IMMUNE SYSTEM RECOGNIZE NEOANTIGENS?

HOW DO NEOANTIGEN VACCINES WORK?

BENEFITS OF NEOANTIGEN CANCER VACCINES

CHALLENGES ASSOCIATED WITH NEOANTIGEN CANCER VACCINES

THINGS PEOPLE SHOULD KNOW ABOUT NEOANTIGEN CANCER VACCINES

CHAPTER 4

THE HISTORY OF NEOANTIGEN CANCER VACCINE RESEARCH

THE EARLY YEARS OF NEOANTIGEN CANCER VACCINE RESEARCH

THE DEVELOPMENT OF PERSONALIZED NEOANTIGEN VACCINES

THE CURRENT STATE OF NEOANTIGEN CANCER VACCINE RESEARCH

THE ETHICAL CONSIDERATIONS OF NEOANTIGEN CANCER VACCINE RESEARCH

CHAPTER 5

IMPACT OF NEOANTIGEN CANCER VACCINE RESEARCH

THE SOCIAL IMPACT OF NEOANTIGEN CANCER VACCINE RESEARCH

THE ECONOMIC IMPACT OF NEOANTIGEN CANCER VACCINE RESEARCH

CHAPTER 6

THE CLINICAL TRIALS OF NEOANTIGEN CANCER VACCINES

THE RESULTS OF EARLY CLINICAL TRIALS

THE RESULTS OF ONGOING CLINICAL TRIALS

THE FUTURE OF CLINICAL TRIALS FOR NEOANTIGEN CANCER VACCINES

THE CHALLENGES AND LIMITATIONS OF NEOANTIGEN CANCER

VACCINES

CHAPTER 7

THE FUTURE OF NEOANTIGEN CANCER VACCINES

ADVANCEMENTS IN NEOANTIGEN PREDICTION AND PERSONALIZATION

COMBINATION THERAPIES AND SYNERGISTIC APPROACHES

OVERCOMING MANUFACTURING AND COST CHALLENGES

EXPANDING APPLICATIONS AND TARGETED INDICATIONS

THE POTENTIAL OF NEOANTIGEN CANCER VACCINES TO

REVOLUTIONIZE CANCER TREATMENT

THE CHALLENGES THAT MUST BE OVERCOME BEFORE NEOANTIGEN

CANCER VACCINES CAN BE WIDELY USED

CHAPTER 8

PATIENT EXPERIENCES

CONCLUSION

INTRODUCTION

Linda was a 45-year-old mother of two who had been feeling run down for months. She chalked it up to the stress of juggling work and family responsibilities, but she knew something was wrong when she started experiencing persistent stomach pain.

Linda made an appointment with her doctor, who ordered a battery of tests. The results were shocking: Linda had stage 4 colon cancer. She was devastated and terrified. She had seen firsthand how devastating cancer could be, as her mother had died from breast cancer when Linda was just 19.

Linda's doctor told her about a new treatment option: a neoantigen cancer vaccine. Linda was hesitant at first, but after researching the treatment and talking to other patients who had tried it, she decided to give it a shot.

The neoantigen cancer vaccine was designed specifically for Linda's unique tumor. The vaccine stimulated her immune system to recognize and attack the cancer cells while leaving healthy cells unharmed.

After several rounds of treatment, Linda's scans showed that her tumors were shrinking. She was elated, and so were her doctors. With the help of the neoantigen cancer vaccine, Linda's cancer was in remission.

Linda's experience underscores the importance of understanding cancer and the latest advances in cancer treatment. Without her knowledge of the neoantigen cancer vaccine, Linda may not have had the chance to fight her cancer in such a targeted and effective way.

The revolution of cancer vaccines is transforming the way we think about cancer treatment. Neoantigen cancer vaccines are personalized, targeted, and offer new hope for patients like Linda. It is crucial for patients and healthcare providers to stay up to date on the latest advancements in cancer treatment to ensure that patients have access to the best possible care.

CHAPTER 1

What is Cancer?

Cancer is a disease that is driven by uncontrolled cell development in the body. These cells can form a tumor, which is a mass of tissue that can grow and spread to other parts of the body. Cancer may begin anywhere in the body, and there are many types of cancer.

The actual cause of cancer is unknown. However, it is likely to result from a combination of hereditary and environmental factors. Some risk factors for cancer include smoking, obesity, exposure to certain chemicals, and a family history of cancer.

There are many different treatments for cancer, including surgery, radiation therapy, chemotherapy, and immunotherapy. The treatment type that is best for a patient depends on the type of cancer, the stage of the cancer, and the patient's overall health.

Cancer is a serious disease, but it is important to remember that many people with cancer can live long and healthy lives. With early detection and treatment, the chances of cancer survival are always improving.

Cancer is the next largest cause of mortality in the United States, behind heart disease. In 2020, there were an estimated 602,350 cancer deaths in the United States. This means that one in four deaths in the United States is due to cancer.

About 1 in 3 people will develop cancer at some point in their lifetime. This means that if you live to be 85, there is a 1 in 3 chance of developing cancer. The likelihood of having cancer rises with age, yet it can afflict people of all ages. However, cancer can affect people of all ages.

Risk Factors for Cancer

Cancer is a complicated disease that can have many different risk factors. Some of the most well-known risk factors for cancer include:

- **Smoking:** Tobacco smoke contains many harmful chemicals that can damage DNA and increase cancer risk. Smoking is a main risk factor for lung cancer and many other types of cancer, such as throat cancer, bladder cancer, and pancreatic cancer.

- **Obesity:** Being overweight or obese can raise the risk of many types of cancer, which include breast cancer, colon cancer, and kidney cancer. One reason for this may be that excess body fat can cause inflammation, which can damage DNA and increase the risk of cancer.

- **Physical inactivity:** Not having enough physical activity can also increase cancer risk. Regular exercise can help keep a healthy weight and reduce inflammation in the body, which may help reduce the risk of cancer.

- **Diet:** A high-processed food diet, red meat, and saturated fat can increase cancer risk. Conversely, a diet high in vegetables, fruits, lean protein, and whole grains can help reduce the risk of cancer.

- **Exposure to certain chemicals:** Exposure to certain chemicals in the workplace or environment can increase the risk of cancer. For example, exposure to asbestos can increase the risk of lung cancer, and exposure to benzene can increase the risk of leukemia.

- **Family history of cancer:** Some types of cancer can run in families. If an individual has a close relative (like parent or sibling) who has had cancer, their own risk of developing that type of cancer may be higher.

- **Certain medical conditions:** Some medical conditions can increase the risk of cancer. For example, people with inflammatory bowel disease (like Crohn's disease or ulcerative colitis) have a higher risk of colon cancer, and people with human papillomavirus (HPV) infection have a higher risk of cervical cancer.

It is important to note that having one or more of these discussed risk factors doesn't necessarily mean a person will develop cancer. Many people who develop cancer do not have any known risk factors, and some individuals who have one or more risk factors never get cancer. However, understanding and managing these risk factors can help reduce cancer risk and promote overall health and well-being.

Cancer Prevention

There are a lot of things that people can do to reduce and prevent the risk of developing cancer. Some of these include:

- **Don't smoke:** Smoking is one of the biggest risk factors for cancer, so avoiding tobacco products (including cigarettes, cigars, and smokeless tobacco) is one of the most necessary things you can do to reduce your risk.

- **Eat a healthy diet:** A diet high in vegetables, fruits, healthy grains, and lean protein can help reduce cancer risk. On the other hand, avoiding those diets that are high in processed-foods, red meat, and saturated fat can increase the risk of cancer.

- **Exercise regularly:** Regular physical activity can help maintain a healthy weight, reduce inflammation in the body, and improve overall health and well-being. This can help reduce the risk of cancer.

- **Maintain a healthy weight:** Being obese or overweight can increase the risk of many types of cancer, so maintaining a healthy weight through a balanced diet and regular exercise is important.

- **Limit your exposure to sunlight:** Excessive exposition to ultraviolet radiation from the sun and tanning booths may raise the risk of skin cancer. To protect your skin, wear protective clothing, use sunscreen with a high SPF, and seek shade during peak sun hours.

- **Get vaccinated against certain viruses, such as the human papillomavirus (HPV):** Certain viruses can increase the risk of cancer, such as HPV (which can increase the risk of cervical, anal, and other types of cancer). Getting vaccinated can help reduce the risk of these types of cancer.

- **Avoid exposure to certain chemicals, such as asbestos and arsenic:** In the workplace or environment, exposure to certain chemicals can increase cancer risk. To reduce this risk, take precautions to avoid exposure to these chemicals whenever possible.

- **Get regular cancer screenings:** Regular screenings can help spot cancer early when it is most treatable. The specific type and frequency of screening tests may vary depending on a person's age, gender, and other risk factors.

In addition to these specific actions, it's also important to put first overall health and well-being by getting enough sleep, managing stress, and avoiding excessive alcohol consumption. By taking these steps, people can help reduce their risk of getting cancer and promote overall health and longevity.

Types of Cancer

Cancer is a category of disorders defined by uncontrolled cell growth and spread throughout the body. There are several types of cancer, each with unique characteristics and symptoms. Understanding the different types of cancer is important in terms of prevention, early detection, and treatment. The most popular types of cancer in the United States are:

- **Lung cancer:** This type of cancer forms in the tissues of the lungs and is commonly caused by smoking. Symptoms involve coughing, shortness of breath, chest pain, and weight loss.

- **Breast cancer:** This cancer begins in the breast cells and is most commonly found in women, but it can also affect men. Symptoms include a thickening or lump in the breast or underarm, changes in breast size, and nipple discharge.

- **Prostate cancer:** This type of cancer develops in the prostate gland in men. Symptoms may include challenges urinating, blood in the semen or urine, and pain in the back, hip, or chest.

- **Colon and rectal cancer:** These cancers develop in the large intestine (colon) or rectum. Symptoms include changes in bowel habits, blood in the stool, abdominal pain, and unintended weight loss.

- **Melanoma:** This is a type of skin cancer that starts in the cells that develop pigment (melanocytes) in the skin. Frequent exposure to ultraviolet (UV) rays from the sun or tanning beds is a common cause. Symptoms include a new mole or change in an existing mole and red, swollen, or painful skin.

- **Non-Hodgkin lymphoma:** This cancer affects the lymphatic system, which is part of the immune system. Symptoms include swollen lymph nodes, fever, and night sweats.

- **Kidney cancer:** This cancer develops in the kidneys, which are in charge of filtering waste products from the blood. Symptoms may include blood in the urine, lower back pain, and a lump in the abdomen.

- **Urinary bladder cancer:** This type of cancer forms in the tissues of the bladder, which stores urine. Symptoms include blood in the urine, pain during urination, and frequent urination.

- **Pancreas cancer:** This cancer develops in the pancreas, an organ behind the stomach that produces enzymes for digestion and hormones that regulate blood sugar. Symptoms include abdominal pain, weight loss, and jaundice (yellowing of the skin and eyes).

- **Thyroid cancer:** This is cancer that originates from the thyroid gland, located in the neck, and is in charge of producing hormones that regulate metabolism. One of the symptoms that may be experienced is the presence of a lump in the neck, difficulty swallowing, and hoarseness.

You must talk to your doctor about your treatment choices if you have been diagnosed with cancer. Many effective treatments are available for cancer, and the chances of survival are always improving.

Cancer is a disease that can afflict anyone, regardless of age. In young adults and children, the most common types of cancer differ from those seen in older adults. Below are the most typical cancer types found in children and young adults:

- **Leukemia:** This cancer affects both the blood and bone marrow. It is the most typical cancer in children and adolescents, contributing to one-third of all cases. Leukemia can cause symptoms such as fatigue, pale skin, fever, and easy bruising or bleeding.

- **Brain tumors:** These can occur in any part of the brain, and the symptoms experienced by an individual will depend on the size and location of the tumor. Symptoms may include headaches, seizures, difficulty with balance or coordination, and changes in vision or hearing.

- **Neuroblastoma:** This cancer develops in nerve cells and can occur anywhere in the body. It is most commonly found in the adrenal glands (located above the kidneys).

Symptoms may include abdominal pain, a mass in the abdomen, and weight loss.

- **Wilms tumor:** This is a form of kidney cancer that is most commonly found in young children. Symptoms may involve abdominal pain, blood in the urine, and a mass in the abdomen.

- **Lymphoma:** This cancer affects the lymphatic system, which is part of the immune system. Lymphoma can be categorized into two main types: Hodgkin lymphoma and non-Hodgkin lymphoma. Symptoms may include swollen lymph nodes, fever, and night sweats.

- **Soft tissue sarcoma:** This cancer type grows in the soft tissues of the body, like muscles, tendons, or fat. Some symptoms may include a lump or swelling in the affected area, pain, and difficulty moving.

- **Rhabdomyosarcoma:** This is a form of soft tissue sarcoma that originates in the muscles attached to bones. It is commonly found in children and can cause symptoms like a lump or swelling, pain, and difficulty moving.

- **Ewing sarcoma:** This is a type of bone cancer usually affects children and young adults. It can cause symptoms such as bone pain, swelling, and a lump or mass in the affected area.

- **Osteosarcoma:** This is another type of bone cancer that usually affects children and young adults. It can cause symptoms such as bone pain, swelling, and difficulty moving the affected limb.

- **Retinoblastoma:** This is a type of eye cancer that usually affects young children. Symptoms may include a white or cloudy appearance in the pupil of the eye, a new squint, and redness or swelling of the eye.

It is important to note that the symptoms of these cancers can be similar to those of other, less serious conditions, so it is important to see a doctor if you or your child is experiencing any concerning symptoms. Early detection and treatment can improve the chances of a successful outcome.

General Signs and Symptoms of Cancer

The signs and symptoms of cancer vary depending on its type and location. Below are some common signs and symptoms to watch out for:

- **Unexplained weight loss:** Losing weight without trying, especially if it is significant, can be a sign of various types of cancer.
- **Fatigue:** Feeling extremely tired and lacking energy, even after getting enough rest, can be a sign of cancer.
- **Pain:** Persistent pain in one part of the body, such as the abdomen, back, or chest, can be a sign of cancer.
- **Skin changes:** Changes in the color, shape, or size of a mole or the development of new spots on the skin can be a sign of skin cancer.

- **Changes in bowel or bladder habits:** Persistent changes in bowel or bladder habits, such as diarrhea, constipation, or blood in the urine or stool, can be a sign of colon, bladder, or prostate cancer.
- **Difficulty swallowing:** Difficulty swallowing or a feeling of something stuck in the throat can be a sign of throat or esophageal cancer.
- **Chronic cough:** A persistent cough that lasts for weeks or months can be a sign of lung cancer.
- **Changes in the menstrual cycle:** Changes in the menstrual cycle, such as heavy bleeding or irregular periods, can signify uterine or cervical cancer.
- **Difficulty urinating:** Difficulty urinating or pain during urination can indicate bladder or prostate cancer.
- **Unexplained fever:** A persistent fever that is not related to an infection can be a sign of

cancer, especially in cases of lymphoma or leukemia.

It is crucial to note that these signs and symptoms can also be caused by other conditions that are not cancer. Still, if you are experiencing any of these symptoms, it is crucial to consult a healthcare provider to determine the underlying cause. Early cancer detection and treatment can significantly improve the chances of successful treatment and cure.

Importance of detecting cancer earlier

Detecting cancer at an earlier stage is crucial for several reasons.

- First and foremost, early detection increases the chances of successful treatment. When cancer is detected early, it is often localized to a specific area and has not spread to other parts of the body. This makes treating it easier with less aggressive and invasive treatment options, such as surgery or radiation therapy. Early detection also increases the chances of a cure, as cancer caught early is more likely to be completely removed or eradicated.

- In addition to improving treatment outcomes, early detection can also save lives. Many types of cancer, like breast, colon, and cervical cancer, can be detected early through screening tests. Regular screenings can aid in detecting cancer in its early periods when it is most treatable. By detecting cancer early and starting treatment promptly, many lives can be saved.

- Another important reason to detect cancer early is that it can reduce the cost of treatment. Advanced cancer often requires more aggressive and expensive treatments, such as chemotherapy and surgery. These treatments can be both physically and emotionally draining and can be a financial burden on patients and their families. By detecting cancer earlier, less invasive and less expensive treatment options can be used, reducing the financial burden on patients and healthcare systems.

- Finally, detecting cancer early can improve the quality of life for patients. Cancer treatment may be both physically and emotionally stressful and can impact patients' ability to work, care for themselves, and enjoy their daily lives. Detecting cancer early can help minimize the impact of treatment on a patient's quality of life, enabling them to go about their everyday activities and maintain their independence.

In summary, detecting cancer earlier is critical for successful treatment, increased chances of a cure, saving lives, reducing the cost of treatment, and improving the quality of life for patients. Regular screenings and early detection can make a significant difference in the outcome of cancer treatment and can ultimately lead to better health outcomes for patients.

Cancer Treatments

There is no one-size-fits-all cure for cancer, but there are many treatments accessible that can help to improve survival rates. There are many different treatments for cancer, and the best treatment for an individual will rely on the type of cancer one have, the stage of cancer, and your overall health.

Some of the most common cancer treatments include:

- **Surgery:** Surgery is a procedure that removes cancer or as much of it as possible. Surgery is often used to treat early-stage cancers.
- **Chemotherapy:** Chemotherapy is a type of treatment that uses drugs to kill cancer cells. Chemotherapy can be given by mouth, injection, or directly into the bloodstream.

- **Radiation therapy:** Radiation therapy makes use of high-energy rays to kill cancer cells. Radiation therapy can be given externally, from a machine outside the body, or internally, by placing radioactive material inside the body.

- **Targeted therapy:** Targeted therapy is a form of treatment that uses drugs to target particular molecules involved in cancer growth. Targeted therapy can be used to treat some types of cancer that are resistant to chemotherapy or radiation therapy.

- **Immunotherapy:** Immunotherapy is a type of treatment that uses the body's own immune system to fight cancer. Immunotherapy can be used to treat some types of cancer that are resistant to other treatments.

Additional to these treatments, there are also many supportive care treatments that can help people with cancer cope with the side effects of treatment and improve their quality of life. Some of the most typical supportive care treatments include:

- **Pain management:** Pain management is important for people with cancer who are experiencing pain. Pain may be caused by the cancer itself, by the treatment, or by both. There are many different ways to manage pain, including medication, physical therapy, and acupuncture.

- **Nutrition:** Nutrition is important for everyone, but it is especially important for people with cancer. Cancer can cause changes in appetite, taste, and digestion, which can make it difficult to eat a healthy diet. There are several resources available to help people with cancer maintain a healthy diet.

- **Fatigue:** Fatigue is a typical side effect of cancer treatment. Fatigue can make it difficult to do daily activities, such as work, exercise, and caring for yourself. There are various things you can do to manage fatigue, such as getting enough sleep, eating a healthy diet, and exercising regularly.

- **Depression:** Depression is a typical side effect of cancer. Depression can make it difficult to cope with the diagnosis, the treatment, and the side effects of treatment. There are a lot of effective treatments for depression, including medication, therapy, and support groups.

- **Anxiety:** Anxiety is another common side effect of cancer. Anxiety can make it difficult to sleep, concentrate, and enjoy life. There are numerous effective treatments for anxiety, including medication, therapy, and support groups.

If you or someone around you has been diagnosed with cancer, you must discuss your treatment options with your doctor. Your doctor can assist you in understanding the risks and benefits of each treatment and choosing the best treatment plan for you.

CHAPTER 2

Cancer vaccine

A cancer vaccine is an immunotherapy that harnesses the body's immune system to fight cancer. Vaccines function by teaching the immune system to recognize and attack a specific disease-causing organism. Cancer vaccines work in a similar way, but they are designed to teach the immune system to recognize and attack cancer cells.

Types of cancer vaccines

Cancer vaccines are a sort of immunotherapy that can help prevent or treat certain types of cancer by boosting the body's immune system to recognize and attack cancer cells. There are two major types of cancer vaccines: preventive vaccines and therapeutic vaccines.

Preventive (prophylactic) vaccines: Preventive vaccines aim to prevent cancer development in the first place. These vaccines can help prevent certain types of cancer caused by infectious agents.

Preventive cancer vaccines are available for some types of cancer, including:

- **Human papillomavirus (HPV) vaccine:** This vaccine protects against the kinds of HPV that can cause cervical cancer, anal cancer, and other types of cancer.
- **Hepatitis B vaccine:** This vaccine protects against hepatitis B, a virus that can cause liver cancer.
- **Hepatitis A vaccine:** This vaccine protects against hepatitis A, a virus that can increase the risk of liver cancer.

- **Human immunodeficiency virus (HIV) vaccine:** Although still in development, this vaccine has the potential to prevent HIV infection, which can elevate the risk of certain types of cancer.

Therapeutic vaccines: Therapeutic vaccines are designed to treat cancer that has already developed.

The purpose of these vaccines is to activate and strengthen the immune system to attack cancer cells already existing in the body. Therapeutic vaccines offer a more targeted approach to cancer treatment than traditional methods such as chemotherapy and radiation. These vaccines aim to specifically attack cancer cells without damaging healthy cells in the process. Some examples of therapeutic cancer vaccines include the sipuleucel-T vaccine for prostate cancer and the pembrolizumab vaccine for melanoma.

Both types of cancer vaccines have shown promise in clinical trials, although much research is still needed to determine their safety and effectiveness. In addition to vaccines specifically designed to prevent or treat cancer, there are also some vaccines that may indirectly help reduce the risk of cancer by preventing other conditions that can increase cancer risk, such as certain types of infections (e.g., HPV, HBV, and the human immunodeficiency virus, or HIV). Overall, cancer vaccines represent an exciting area of research and development in the fight against cancer.

There are a few things that people should know about cancer vaccines:

1. They are not a cure for cancer, but they can help slow the tumor's growth or even lead to remission.
2. They can cause some side effects, such as fatigue, fever, and chills.

3. They are not yet widely available, but they are becoming more common as the technology improves.

4. They can be expensive, but there are some financial assistance programs available.

If you're interested in gaining further knowledge about cancer vaccines, talk to your doctor. They can help you determine if this type of immunotherapy is right for you.

The Evolution of Cancer Vaccines

The development of cancer vaccines has undergone a remarkable evolution over the years, with significant advancements in understanding tumor immunology and the role of neoantigens. In this chapter, we will explore the history of cancer vaccines and how the discovery of neoantigens has transformed the field, leading to personalized and targeted immunotherapy options.

Early Attempts at Cancer Vaccines

The early years: This section delves into the initial attempts at developing cancer vaccines, dating back to the late 19th century. It explores pioneering research by William Coley and his use of bacterial toxins to induce immune responses against tumors, marking the foundation of cancer immunotherapy.

The era of tumor-associated antigens: Here, we explore the identification and utilization of tumor-associated antigens (TAAs) as targets for cancer vaccines. The discovery of specific antigens expressed by cancer cells led to efforts to develop vaccines to stimulate immune responses against these antigens.

The Emergence of Neoantigens

Neoantigens: A paradigm shift: This section focuses on the groundbreaking discovery of neoantigens, marking a significant turning point in cancer vaccine development. The concept of neoantigens, unique markers arising from genetic mutations in cancer cells, brought personalized medicine to the forefront of cancer immunotherapy.

Advances in genomic sequencing: The advent of high-throughput sequencing technologies enabled the identification and characterization of neoantigens on a genomic scale. This breakthrough allowed researchers to unravel the genetic landscape of tumors and pinpoint neoantigens specific to individual patients.

The Neoantigen Revolution in Cancer Vaccines

Personalized neoantigen vaccines: This section highlights the development of personalized neoantigen vaccines that harness the unique genetic makeup of an individual's tumor. By identifying patient-specific neoantigens, these vaccines stimulate an immune response precisely tailored to target and eliminate cancer cells.

Adoptive cell therapies and neoantigens: Here, we explore the integration of neoantigens into adoptive cell therapies, such as CAR-T cell therapy and TIL therapy. Neoantigen-specific T cells can be engineered or isolated from the patient's own immune cells, providing a potent and targeted immunotherapy approach.

Future of Cancer Vaccines

Advancements in neoantigen prediction: This section discusses the ongoing advancements in bioinformatics algorithms and machine learning techniques to improve the prediction of neoantigens. These advancements will enable more accurate and efficient identification of neoantigens, further enhancing the efficacy of cancer vaccines.

Combination therapies and synergistic approaches: The future of cancer vaccines lies in their integration with other treatment modalities, such as immune checkpoint inhibitors, targeted therapies, and traditional chemotherapy. This section explores the potential synergistic effects of combining cancer vaccines with other treatments to achieve optimal outcomes.

The evolution of cancer vaccines has witnessed significant milestones, from early attempts at stimulating immune responses against tumors to the emergence of personalized neoantigen vaccines. The concept of neoantigens has revolutionized the field, bringing about a paradigm shift towards personalized and targeted immunotherapy. As research and technological advancements continue, the future of cancer vaccines holds great promise for improving patient outcomes and transforming the cancer treatment landscape.

Neoantigen Cancer Vaccine

CHAPTER 3

The Science Behind

Neoantigens

Neoantigens, a term coined in the field of cancer immunology, play a crucial role in the development of personalized cancer therapies. These unique molecular markers are derived from genetic mutations that occur within cancer cells. Understanding the science behind neoantigens is key to unlocking their potential for targeted immunotherapy and revolutionizing cancer treatment. Understanding the biology of neoantigens and their interaction with the immune system enables the development of personalized cancer therapies that hold great promise for improving treatment outcomes and revolutionizing the field of oncology.

Introduction to Neoantigen Cancer Vaccines
Neoantigen cancer vaccines are a new type of immunotherapy that is designed to train the body's immune system to fight cancer. Neoantigens are proteins that are created when cancer cells mutate. These mutations can make cancer cells look different from normal cells, which can help the immune system to recognize and attack them.

Neoantigen cancer vaccines work by delivering neoantigens to the body's immune system. This can be done in different ways, including injecting the neoantigens directly into the body or using nanoparticles to deliver the neoantigens to the immune system. Once the neoantigens are in the body, they can stimulate the immune system to produce T cells that are specifically targeted to the cancer cells.

Neoantigen cancer vaccines are a promising new approach to cancer treatment. They have the potential to improve cancer survival rates, reduce the cost of cancer treatment, and make cancer treatment more accessible. Despite the potential benefits, some challenges still need to be resolved before neoantigen cancer vaccines can be widely adopted. These challenges include the cost of neoantigen cancer vaccines, the complexity of manufacturing neoantigen cancer vaccines, and the difficulty of identifying neoantigens that are recognized by the immune system. Despite these challenges, neoantigen cancer vaccines represent a promising new hope for cancer patients.

What are neoantigens?

Imagine a key that unlocks the body's defense system against cancer. This key is known as a neoantigen. A neoantigen is a protein that is produced when a mutation occurs in a gene. Neoantigens are proteins found on the surface of cancer cells that differentiate them from normal cells. They arise from genetic mutations or alterations within the tumor, making them unique to each individual and their specific cancer. These specific proteins hold the potential to trigger a powerful immune response, leading to the destruction of cancer cells.

How are neoantigens generated?

Neoantigens are generated through a complex interplay of genetic mutations and tumor-specific alterations. When a cell undergoes mutations, changes occur in its DNA, which can result from environmental factors, such as exposure to carcinogens or errors during DNA replication. These mutations can produce abnormal proteins, including neoantigens, which act as beacons for the immune system.

These changes can make the cancer cells look different from normal cells, which can help the immune system to recognize and attack them.

How does the immune system recognize neoantigens?

The immune system can recognize neoantigens through a process called antigen presentation. In antigen presentation, dendritic cells (DCs) take up neoantigens from cancer cells and present them to T cells. T cells are a form of white blood cell that is responsible for fighting infection. When T cells see neoantigens, they can become activated and start to attack the cancer cells.

The immune system's ability to identify and eliminate cancer cells is vital in combating the disease. Neoantigens play a critical role in this process. Specialized immune cells, such as T cells, patrol the body in search of foreign invaders or abnormal cells. These T cells possess receptors called T cell receptors (TCRs), which can recognize and bind to specific neoantigens presented on the surface of cancer cells. Once bound, T cells initiate an immune response against the cancerous cells.

How do neoantigen vaccines work?

Neoantigen vaccines work by delivering neoantigens to the body's immune system. This can be done in different ways, including injecting the neoantigens directly into the body or using nanoparticles to deliver the neoantigens to the immune system. Once the neoantigens are in the body, they can stimulate the immune system to produce T cells that are specifically targeted at the cancer cells.

Neoantigen vaccines represent a revolutionary approach to cancer immunotherapy. They make use of the power of the immune system to specifically target and eliminate cancer cells bearing neoantigens. The process begins by analyzing the patient's tumor through genetic sequencing and computational algorithms to identify the unique neoantigens present. This personalized information is then used to create a customized vaccine.

The neoantigen vaccine consists of synthetic neoantigens derived from the patient's tumor, which are combined with an adjuvant. The adjuvant serves as a stimulator, enhancing the immune response triggered by the vaccine. When administered to the patient, the vaccine acts as a "training manual" for the immune system, providing instructions on recognizing and attacking the cancer cells.

Upon vaccination, the immune system receives a potent stimulus to recognize the neoantigens as foreign and mount a targeted immune response. The T cells, armed with the information from the vaccine, are activated to seek out and destroy cancer cells presenting the specific neoantigens. This approach aims to generate a robust and durable immune response against cancer, potentially leading to tumor regression or elimination.

Neoantigen vaccines are still undergoing extensive research and clinical trials, with promising early results suggesting their efficacy in certain types of cancer. As research progresses, these vaccines hold the potential to revolutionize cancer treatment by offering a personalized, targeted, and immunologically-based approach to combating the disease.

This chapter lays the foundation for understanding the significance of neoantigens, their generation, and their recognition by the immune system. It also provides an overview of how neoantigen vaccines harness the body's immune response to fight cancer. As we delve deeper into subsequent chapters, we will explore the development, challenges, and future prospects of neoantigen cancer vaccines, ultimately aiming to unlock new frontiers in cancer treatment.

Benefits of Neoantigen cancer vaccines

Neoantigen cancer vaccines are a promising new treatment for cancer. They have the potential to improve the outcomes of patients with cancer by stimulating the body's immune system to fight cancer cells.

Here are some of the benefits of neoantigen cancer vaccines:

- **Personalized therapy:** Neoantigen cancer vaccines are tailored to the individual patient, meaning that each vaccine is unique and designed specifically to target the patient's cancer cells. This personalized approach could potentially enhance treatment outcomes and reduce side effects compared to traditional therapies.

- **Targeted therapy:** Neoantigen cancer vaccines target only the cancer cells and spare healthy tissue, reducing the risk of side effects such as nausea, hair loss, and fatigue associated with chemotherapy and radiation therapy.

- **Durability of response:** Neoantigen cancer vaccines have the potential to induce long-lasting immune responses that can continue to attack cancer cells even after the initial treatment is completed. This is because the immune system has a "memory" of the cancer cells and can recognize and attack them if they reappear.

- **Broader applicability:** Neoantigen cancer vaccines have the potential to treat a broad range of cancers, including those that are resistant to traditional therapies. This is because neoantigens are unique to each patient's cancer cells, meaning that the therapy can be tailored to the specific characteristics of each tumor.

- **Combinatorial potential:** Neoantigen cancer vaccines can be combined with other immunotherapies or traditional therapies to enhance their effectiveness. For example, combining a neoantigen cancer vaccine with an immune checkpoint inhibitor has been shown to improve outcomes in certain types of cancer.

Overall, the development of neoantigen cancer vaccines represents an exciting new area of cancer research that has the potential to transform cancer treatment and improve outcomes for patients. Ongoing clinical trials are currently evaluating the safety and effectiveness of these therapies, and further research is required to properly understand the potential benefits and limitations of this approach.

Challenges associated with Neoantigen cancer vaccines

Neoantigen cancer vaccines are a promising area of cancer research that involves using the body's own immune system to notice and attack cancer cells. Neoantigens are unique proteins that are present on the surface of cancer cells but not on normal cells, making them an ideal target for immunotherapy. However, there are several challenges associated with developing effective neoantigen cancer vaccines, including:

- **Identifying the right neoantigens:** Identifying the specific neoantigens that are present in a patient's cancer cells can be challenging, as these proteins can vary from patient to patient and even from one cancer cell to another within the same patient. Researchers must use sophisticated bioinformatics tools to analyze cancer cells and identify the neoantigens that are most likely to be recognized by the immune system.

- **Overcoming tumor heterogeneity:** Even within a single tumor, there can be significant heterogeneity, meaning that different cells within the tumor can have different neoantigens. This can make it difficult to develop a vaccine that can effectively target all the cancer cells.

- **Stimulating a strong immune response:** Cancer cells are often able to defeat the immune system by suppressing the immune response or by expressing immune checkpoint molecules that inhibit T cell activation. A major challenge is developing a vaccine that can stimulate a strong and sustained immune response against cancer cells.

- **Manufacturing challenges:** Neoantigen cancer vaccines are personalized therapies that are tailored to each individual patient. This means that each vaccine must be manufactured on a case-by-case basis, which can be time-consuming and expensive.

- **Regulatory challenges:** The development and approval of neoantigen cancer vaccines can be challenging due to the complex nature of the therapy and the need for individualized manufacturing. Regulatory agencies must ensure that these therapies are safe and effective while also balancing the need for timely approval with the need for a thorough evaluation.

Despite these challenges, neoantigen cancer vaccines hold great promise as a potentially curative therapy for certain types of cancer. Ongoing research is focused on addressing these challenges and improving the effectiveness of these innovative therapies.

Things people should know about neoantigen cancer vaccines

Here are some important things that people should know about neoantigen cancer vaccines:

- **Neoantigen cancer vaccines are a type of immunotherapy:** Neoantigen cancer vaccines are a type of cancer treatment that leverages the power of the body's own immune system to recognize and attack cancer cells. They are part of a broader class of treatments known as immunotherapies, which also include immune checkpoint inhibitors and CAR-T cell therapies.

- **They are personalized:** Neoantigen cancer vaccines are tailored to the individual patient, meaning that each vaccine is unique and designed specifically to target the patient's cancer cells. This is because neoantigens are unique to each patient's tumor, so the vaccine must be tailored to the specific characteristics of each tumor.

- **They are still experimental:** Neoantigen cancer vaccines are a relatively new area of cancer research, and there is still much unknown information regarding their safety and effectiveness. Clinical trials are ongoing, and the long-term outcomes of these therapies are not yet clear.

- **They are not a cure-all:** While neoantigen cancer vaccines have shown promise in early clinical trials, they are not a cure-all for cancer. They may be effective in certain types of cancer but not in others, and they may not work for everyone.

- **They have potential side effects:** Neoantigen cancer vaccines can have side effects like all cancer treatments. These may include fatigue, fever, chills, headaches, and muscle aches. However, the side effects of neoantigen cancer vaccines are generally milder than those of traditional chemotherapy and radiation therapy.

- **They are not yet widely available:** The development of neoantigen cancer vaccines is still in its early stages and is not yet widely available. However, as clinical trials continue and more research is conducted, it is possible that these therapies will become more easily accessible in the future.

Overall, neoantigen cancer vaccines are an exciting new area of cancer research that can potentially transform cancer treatment. However, it is important to approach these therapies cautiously and work closely with your healthcare provider to determine whether they are an appropriate treatment option for you.

Neoantigen Cancer Vaccine

CHAPTER 4

The History of Neoantigen

Cancer Vaccine Research

Over the years, the field of cancer research has witnessed tremendous progress, leading to the development of innovative therapies and treatments. Among these groundbreaking approaches, neoantigen cancer vaccines have emerged as a promising frontier in the fight against cancer. By harnessing the power of personalized immunotherapy, neoantigen cancer vaccines aim to unleash the potential of the human immune system to specifically target and eradicate cancer cells.

The history of neoantigen cancer vaccine research is a captivating tale of scientific exploration, perseverance, and the relentless pursuit of new treatment modalities. It traces back to the discovery of neoantigens, unique proteins that adorn the surface of cancer cells, setting them apart from healthy cells within the body.

Early investigations into neoantigens revealed their potential as key players in the immune system's recognition and targeting of cancer cells. Researchers recognized that these neoantigens could serve as specific markers, enabling the immune system to identify and attack cancerous growths while sparing normal, healthy tissue.

The advent of genomic sequencing technologies provided a crucial turning point in neoantigen cancer vaccine research. These tools allowed scientists to delve deep into the genetic makeup of tumors, identifying the specific mutations and alterations that give rise to neoantigens. By deciphering the complex genomic landscape of cancer cells, researchers gained valuable insights into the unique neoantigens present in each individual's tumor, paving the way for personalized vaccine development.

In recent years, pioneering studies and clinical trials have showcased the potential of neoantigen cancer vaccines in eliciting robust and targeted immune responses against cancer. These early successes have fueled an exponential growth in research, attracting the attention and collaboration of scientists, clinicians, and pharmaceutical companies worldwide.

However, challenges remain on the path to realizing the full potential of neoantigen cancer vaccines. The development of personalized vaccines requires intricate processes, from identifying neoantigens to designing and manufacturing individualized vaccines for each patient. Additionally, optimizing the delivery and efficacy of these vaccines poses further complexities that researchers strive to overcome.

As the history of neoantigen cancer vaccine research continues to unfold, the promise of personalized immunotherapy as a transformative approach to cancer treatment becomes increasingly tangible. With ongoing advancements in genomics, computational biology, and immunology, researchers are pushing the boundaries of our understanding and capabilities, inching closer to a future where neoantigen cancer vaccines may offer new avenues of hope and healing for patients facing this formidable disease.

The Early Years of Neoantigen Cancer Vaccine Research

The effort to harness the power of the immune system against cancer has been a long and challenging journey. The concept of neoantigens as key targets for immunotherapy emerged from the understanding that cancer cells bear unique protein markers that differentiate them from healthy cells. The notion of personalized neoantigen cancer vaccines began to take shape as researchers recognized the potential of these specific antigens in triggering an effective immune response against tumors.

In the early years of neoantigen cancer vaccine research, scientists focused on understanding the fundamental biology of neoantigens and their role in cancer development. The advent of genomic sequencing technologies and advances in bioinformatics played a pivotal role in this exploration. Researchers could now identify and characterize the genetic mutations that give rise to neoantigens, paving the way for their utilization in vaccine design.

The Development of Personalized Neoantigen Vaccines

The development of personalized neoantigen vaccines marked a significant milestone in cancer immunotherapy. Recognizing that each patient's cancer is unique, researchers realized the importance of tailoring vaccines to target the specific neoantigens present in an individual's tumor. This approach aimed to enhance the vaccine's effectiveness by ensuring a personalized immune response against the cancer cells.

With the rapid advancements in genomic sequencing and computational tools, researchers can now analyze the genetic makeup of tumors and identify the neoantigens within them. This information enabled the design and synthesis of personalized neoantigen vaccines comprising a selection of patient-specific neoantigens. These vaccines were combined with adjuvants to enhance immune activation and administered to patients, triggering an immune response specifically targeted against their unique cancer cells.

The development of personalized neoantigen vaccines presented significant challenges, including the complexity and cost associated with analyzing tumor genomes, identifying relevant neoantigens, and manufacturing individualized vaccines. However, the potential benefits of these vaccines, including improved efficacy and reduced toxicity, fueled ongoing research and propelled the field forward.

The Current State of Neoantigen Cancer Vaccine Research

The current state of neoantigen cancer vaccine research is marked by remarkable progress and increasing optimism. Clinical trials have demonstrated the potential of personalized neoantigen vaccines to elicit robust immune responses and induce tumor regression in specific cancer types.

Ongoing research is focused on refining vaccine design and delivery strategies, optimizing immune activation, and overcoming challenges associated with neoantigen identification and manufacturing. Advances in technologies such as machine learning, artificial intelligence, and high-throughput sequencing are facilitating the identification of neoantigens more efficiently and accurately, thus streamlining the vaccine development process.

Collaborations between academia, industry, and regulatory agencies have further accelerated the translation of neoantigen cancer vaccines from the lab to clinical practice. The regulatory landscape is evolving to accommodate the unique nature of personalized vaccines, ensuring that rigorous standards are met while enabling timely development and access to these innovative treatments.

While challenges remain, the remarkable progress in neoantigen cancer vaccine research has generated excitement and renewed hope in the fight against cancer. The potential of personalized vaccines to revolutionize cancer treatment by leveraging the body's immune system underscores the significance of ongoing research efforts. It provides a beacon of hope for patients and healthcare providers alike.

This chapter has shed light on the historical trajectory of neoantigen cancer vaccine research, from its early foundations to the current state of the field. In the following chapters, we will explore milestones, challenges, and recent breakthroughs in neoantigen cancer vaccine research. By examining the rich tapestry of scientific achievements and the collaborative efforts of dedicated professionals, we can grasp the immense potential of this innovative approach and anticipate the exciting possibilities it holds for the future of cancer treatment.

The Ethical Considerations of Neoantigen Cancer Vaccine Research

Neoantigen cancer vaccine research holds great promise in revolutionizing cancer treatment by leveraging the body's immune system to target and eliminate cancer cells. However, along with its potential benefits, this innovative field of research raises important ethical considerations that need careful attention.

This chapter will explore the ethical considerations surrounding neoantigen cancer vaccine research. We will delve into the right to privacy and the protection of patients' personal genetic information. We will also discuss the significance of informed consent, ensuring that patients clearly understand the research process and potential risks. Additionally, we will address the risk of adverse side effects and the responsibility of researchers in ensuring patient safety.

By critically examining these ethical dimensions, we can navigate the challenges and complexities that arise in neoantigen cancer vaccine research. Ethical integrity, patient autonomy, and safeguarding patient well-being are central to the responsible advancement of this groundbreaking field. Through thoughtful consideration of these ethical considerations, we can strive towards conducting scientifically sound and ethically robust research.

The Right to Privacy

Neoantigen cancer vaccine research involves collecting and analyzing personal genetic information from patients. This raises important ethical considerations regarding the right to privacy. Patients have the right to control and protect their personal health information, including their genomic data. Researchers must ensure the confidentiality and security of this sensitive information to safeguard patient privacy.

Strict adherence to data protection regulations and ethical guidelines is essential when handling genomic data. Robust measures should be implemented to prevent unauthorized access, use, or disclosure of patient information. Transparent communication with patients regarding data privacy policies and obtaining informed consent for data sharing is crucial to upholding their rights and fostering trust in the research process.

The Right to Informed Consent

Respecting patient autonomy and ensuring informed consent is paramount in neoantigen cancer vaccine research. Patients must be provided with comprehensive information about the research, including the purpose, potential risks and benefits, alternatives, and the implications of participating or declining participation. Informed consent should be obtained voluntarily, without coercion, and based on a thorough understanding of the information provided.

Patients should be informed about the possible consequences of sharing their genomic and medical data due to the personalized nature of neoantigen cancer vaccines. Clear communication should address the possibility of incidental findings, which are unexpected genetic findings unrelated to cancer but may have implications for the patient's health. Patients must be given the opportunity to ask questions, seek clarification, and make an informed decision about their participation.

The Risk of Adverse Side Effects

Like any medical intervention, neoantigen cancer vaccines carry the potential for adverse side effects. Ethical considerations arise in ensuring patient safety and minimizing risks while conducting research. Researchers are responsible for thoroughly evaluating the vaccine's safety profile and mitigating potential harm.

Prior to initiating clinical trials, preclinical studies should provide robust evidence of safety and efficacy in relevant animal models. Comprehensive monitoring and reporting of adverse events during clinical trials are essential to promptly detecting and managing any potential side effects. Open and transparent communication with patients regarding known risks, potential side effects, and the steps taken to mitigate them is crucial in maintaining trust and obtaining informed consent.

Furthermore, researchers should prioritize the long-term monitoring and follow-up of patients after vaccination to identify any delayed or rare adverse effects that may emerge. This ongoing vigilance ensures patient safety and contributes to the continuous evaluation and improvement of neoantigen cancer vaccine research.

This chapter has explored the ethical considerations surrounding neoantigen cancer vaccine research. Upholding the right to privacy, obtaining informed consent, and managing the risk of adverse side effects are crucial aspects of conducting ethically sound research. By addressing these considerations with diligence and respect, researchers can foster trust, protect patient autonomy, and contribute to the responsible advancement of neoantigen cancer vaccines.

CHAPTER 5

Impact of Neoantigen Cancer Vaccine Research

Neoantigen cancer vaccine research represents a paradigm shift in the field of cancer treatment, offering new hope and possibilities in the fight against this devastating disease. The potential impact of these innovative vaccines reaches far beyond the realms of science and medicine, touching upon various aspects of healthcare, society, and the economy.

In this chapter, we will explore the multifaceted impact of neoantigen cancer vaccine research. We will delve into these vaccines' potential benefits, including improved patient outcomes, reduced healthcare costs, and enhanced accessibility to effective treatments. Additionally, we will examine the social and economic implications, such as job creation, industry growth, and advancements in healthcare infrastructure.

The impact of neoantigen cancer vaccine research extends beyond the individual level and has the potential to transform the landscape of cancer care. By leveraging the body's immune system to target cancer cells based on their specific genetic mutations, these vaccines have the potential to revolutionize treatment approaches and improve survival rates.

Moreover, the impact of these vaccines resonates within society, addressing ethical considerations, such as privacy and informed consent, and promoting equitable access to advanced therapies. Additionally, the economic implications of neoantigen cancer vaccine research cannot be overlooked, as it has the potential to create new job opportunities, stimulate industry growth, and contribute to healthcare system sustainability.

As we navigate this chapter, we must recognize the transformative power of neoantigen cancer vaccine research. By understanding and harnessing the impact, we can drive positive change in healthcare delivery, improve patient experiences, and ultimately work towards a future where effective and personalized treatments are accessible to all individuals affected by cancer.

In the subsequent sections, we will explore further the specific dimensions of impact, exploring the potential benefits, challenges, and opportunities associated with neoantigen cancer vaccine research. By doing so, we aim to illuminate the full extent of the impact and empower stakeholders to make informed decisions that will shape the future of cancer treatment.

Let us now explore the impact of neoantigen cancer vaccine research, where scientific advancement intersects with social progress and economic prosperity.

The Social Impact of Neoantigen Cancer Vaccine Research

Neoantigen cancer vaccine research holds not only significant potential in advancing cancer treatment but also carries substantial social implications. The creation and use of these vaccines could completely change how cancer is treated and greatly impact the health of people, communities, and society overall.

In this section, we will explore the social impact of neoantigen cancer vaccine research. We will examine how these vaccines can enhance patient outcomes and quality of life by offering more targeted and personalized treatment options. We will also discuss the potential economic implications of these vaccines, considering factors such as healthcare costs, accessibility, and equity.

Furthermore, we will delve into the societal implications of neoantigen cancer vaccine research, including its impact on healthcare systems, research infrastructure, and policy considerations. We will discuss the challenges and opportunities associated with integrating these innovative therapies into existing healthcare frameworks and the potential for fostering collaboration between various stakeholders.

Understanding the social impact of neoantigen cancer vaccine research is essential for promoting responsible and equitable implementation. By exploring these dimensions, we can assess the potential benefits and risks, address disparities in access and affordability, and shape policies that ensure equitable distribution and maximize societal benefits.

As we embark on this exploration, it is crucial to recognize the transformative potential of neoantigen cancer vaccines and the importance of considering the broader social implications beyond the realm of scientific advancement. By carefully evaluating the social impact, we can strive to harness the full potential of these vaccines to improve cancer care and positively influence the well-being of people and society as a whole.

The Potential to Improve Cancer Survival Rates

Neoantigen cancer vaccine research has the potential to significantly impact cancer survival rates. By leveraging the body's immune system to target and eliminate cancer cells, these vaccines offer a personalized and targeted approach to cancer treatment. This individualized approach can enhance treatment efficacy and improve patient outcomes.

Neoantigen vaccines, tailored to the specific genetic mutations present in a patient's tumor, have shown promise in clinical trials. They stimulate a robust and targeted immune response against cancer cells bearing neoantigens, leading to tumor regression and prolonged survival. With further research and advancements in vaccine design, these therapies have the potential to improve overall cancer survival rates, offering hope to patients and their families.

The Potential to Reduce the Cost of Cancer Treatment

The financial burden associated with cancer treatment is a significant concern for patients, families, and healthcare systems. Neoantigen cancer vaccines have the potential to reduce the cost of cancer treatment in several ways.

Firstly, the personalized nature of neoantigen vaccines enables a more targeted approach, minimizing the need for broad-spectrum treatments with potential side effects and associated costs. By specifically targeting cancer cells bearing neoantigens, these vaccines can potentially reduce the use of costly treatments that may not be effective or necessary for each patient.

Secondly, the development of neoantigen cancer vaccines could lead to increased competition in the pharmaceutical industry, potentially driving down the overall cost of cancer treatment. As more companies and researchers enter the field, the availability and affordability of these therapies may improve, benefiting patients and healthcare systems alike.

The Potential to Make Cancer Treatment More Accessible

One of the significant challenges in cancer treatment is ensuring equitable access to effective therapies. Neoantigen cancer vaccines have the potential to address this issue by making cancer treatment more accessible.

Personalized neoantigen vaccines can be tailored to the unique genetic makeup of each patient's tumor, allowing for a customized treatment approach. This individualized strategy could benefit patients who may not respond well to conventional therapies or have limited treatment options. By expanding the range of available treatments, neoantigen cancer vaccines have the potential to provide hope and improved outcomes for individuals who may have otherwise faced limited treatment options.

Additionally, the development of neoantigen vaccines has the potential to foster collaborations between academic institutions, pharmaceutical companies, and healthcare providers. Such collaborations can facilitate sharing of knowledge, resources, and technologies, leading to advancements in vaccine development and increased accessibility to these innovative therapies.

By addressing the social impact of neoantigen cancer vaccine research, we can envision a future where cancer survival rates improve, treatment costs decrease, and access to effective therapies becomes more equitable. The transformative potential of these vaccines extends beyond the realm of scientific advancement, offering hope and positively influencing the lives of individuals, communities, and society as a whole.

In this section, we have explored the potential of neoantigen cancer vaccines to improve cancer survival rates, reduce the cost of treatment, and make cancer treatment more accessible. Addressing the challenges and opportunities associated with these vaccines is crucial as we move forward, ensuring their responsible integration into healthcare systems and realizing their full societal benefits.

The Economic Impact of Neoantigen Cancer Vaccine Research

Neoantigen cancer vaccine research has the potential to bring about significant economic implications in the field of cancer treatment and healthcare at large. As these innovative vaccines continue to advance, it becomes crucial to examine their economic impact from multiple angles, including healthcare costs, industry growth, and resource allocation.

In this section, we will explore the economic impact of neoantigen cancer vaccine research. We will delve into how these vaccines have the potential to shape healthcare costs by offering more targeted and personalized treatment options. Additionally, we will examine the economic implications for the pharmaceutical industry, exploring the potential for growth and investment in this burgeoning field. Moreover, we will discuss resource allocation considerations and the challenges associated with integrating neoantigen vaccines into existing healthcare systems.

By understanding the economic impact of neoantigen cancer vaccine research, we can evaluate the potential benefits and challenges that arise. This understanding can inform policy decisions, healthcare resource allocation, and investment strategies to ensure that the economic implications align with the broader goals of improving patient outcomes, reducing healthcare costs, and fostering sustainable healthcare systems.

As we embark on this exploration, it is crucial to recognize that the economic impact of neoantigen cancer vaccine research extends beyond immediate financial considerations. The economic implications can influence access to innovative therapies, drive research and development, and shape the overall landscape of cancer treatment. By critically examining these dimensions, we can foster an environment that promotes responsible economic growth and maximizes the societal benefits of neoantigen cancer vaccine research.

The Potential to Create New Jobs in the Healthcare Industry

Neoantigen cancer vaccine research has the potential to create new job opportunities within the healthcare industry. As this field continues to advance, the demand for specialized professionals such as geneticists, immunologists, bioinformaticians, and clinical researchers will likely increase. Developing, producing, and administering neoantigen vaccines require a multidisciplinary team, leading to job growth in various healthcare sectors.

Furthermore, as the field expands, there may be a need for additional healthcare infrastructure, such as specialized clinics or research centers, to accommodate the demand for neoantigen cancer vaccine research and treatment. These facilities would create job opportunities for healthcare providers, support staff, and administrative personnel, further contributing to employment growth.

The creation of new jobs in the healthcare industry supports economic growth and enhances the capacity to provide quality care and support to cancer patients. By fostering job opportunities, neoantigen cancer vaccine research can positively impact the workforce and improve communities' overall health and well-being.

The Potential to Generate New Revenue for the Healthcare Industry

Neoantigen cancer vaccine research has the potential to generate new revenue streams for the healthcare industry. Developing and commercializing these vaccines can open up opportunities for pharmaceutical companies, biotech firms, and research institutions to invest in innovative therapies. This investment can lead to the development of new drugs, diagnostic tools, and treatment technologies, resulting in increased revenue for these industries.

Additionally, the adoption of neoantigen cancer vaccines can drive demand for supportive services and infrastructure. This includes diagnostic testing, patient monitoring, and follow-up care, which can contribute to the growth of ancillary healthcare services and generate revenue for healthcare providers.

Moreover, the economic benefits extend beyond the immediate healthcare sector. The development of neoantigen cancer vaccines can attract investments, spur innovation, and foster collaborations within the broader life sciences industry. This interplay between various sectors can result in economic growth, job creation, and technological advancements, with ripple effects throughout the economy.

The Possibility to Enhance the Quality of Life for Cancer Patients

Research on neoantigen cancer vaccines has an important economic impact in improving the quality of life for cancer patients. By offering more targeted and personalized treatment options, these vaccines have the potential to enhance patient outcomes and well-being.

Neoantigen cancer vaccines can reduce the reliance on conventional, broad-spectrum treatments that often come with significant side effects. This personalized approach minimizes unnecessary treatment-related discomfort, improving patients' quality of life. Moreover, by effectively targeting cancer cells, these vaccines can enhance treatment efficacy, potentially resulting in better disease control and improved overall patient well-being.

Furthermore, the economic impact extends to cancer care's social and psychological aspects. Improved treatment outcomes and reduced treatment burdens can alleviate financial stress and emotional strain for patients and their families. This improved quality of life can positively impact productivity, social engagement, and overall societal well-being.

In summary, this chapter has explored the economic impact of neoantigen cancer vaccine research. This field has the potential to create new job opportunities, generate revenue, and improve the quality of life for cancer patients, which showcases its significant impact. By considering these economic dimensions, stakeholders can make informed decisions, develop supportive policies, and invest in the responsible advancement of neoantigen cancer vaccines, fostering a thriving healthcare industry and benefiting patients and society.

CHAPTER 6

The Clinical Trials of

Neoantigen Cancer Vaccines

Clinical trials play a crucial role in developing and evaluating neoantigen cancer vaccines, paving the way for their eventual approval and widespread use in cancer treatment. These trials provide a rigorous and systematic approach to assessing these innovative vaccines' safety, efficacy, and potential side effects in human subjects.

This chapter will delve into the realm of clinical trials for neoantigen cancer vaccines. We will explore the significance of these trials in advancing our understanding of these therapies and ensuring their effectiveness in real-world settings. From early-phase trials assessing safety and dosage to late-phase trials examining long-term outcomes, these studies are essential for establishing neoantigen cancer vaccines' validity and therapeutic potential.

We will discuss the various phases of clinical trials, from preclinical research to large-scale randomized controlled trials, shedding light on the rigorous processes involved in assessing the safety and efficacy of these vaccines. Additionally, we will explore the challenges and considerations unique to neoantigen cancer vaccine trials, such as the personalized nature of the treatment, patient selection criteria, and the importance of biomarker identification.

By conducting well-designed and meticulously executed clinical trials, researchers aim to gather robust evidence regarding the benefits and limitations of neoantigen cancer vaccines. This evidence is essential for regulatory authorities, healthcare professionals, and patients to make informed decisions regarding the integration of these vaccines into standard cancer treatment protocols.

The outcomes of these trials have the potential to reshape the landscape of cancer care, offering more targeted and personalized treatment options that harness the power of the immune system. Additionally, the knowledge gained from these trials contributes to the broader understanding of immunotherapy and paves the way for future advancements in cancer treatment.

As we explore the clinical trials of neoantigen cancer vaccines, it is crucial to recognize the critical role that research participants, healthcare professionals, and regulatory agencies play in advancing the field. By diligently following ethical guidelines and scientific rigor, clinical trials provide the evidence base necessary for the responsible integration of neoantigen cancer vaccines into clinical practice, ultimately benefiting cancer patients worldwide.

Now, we will explore the realm of clinical trials in more detail, where scientific discovery meets human determination in the pursuit of improved cancer treatment and better patient outcomes.

The Results of Early Clinical Trials

Early clinical trials evaluating neoantigen cancer vaccines have yielded promising results, offering hope for the future of cancer treatment. These initial studies focused on assessing the safety, feasibility, and immunogenicity of these personalized vaccines in small cohorts of patients.

In one study, patients with advanced melanoma who received a neoantigen vaccine had a median survival time of 20 months, compared to 12 months for patients who received standard-of-care treatment. In another study, patients with advanced colorectal cancer who received a neoantigen vaccine had a median progression-free survival time of 10 months, compared to 5 months for patients who received standard-of-care treatment.

The results of early clinical trials have demonstrated that neoantigen cancer vaccines can elicit potent immune responses specifically targeting cancer cells bearing neoantigens. These vaccines have shown favorable safety profiles, with limited adverse effects reported. Moreover, preliminary evidence suggests that neoantigen vaccines can lead to tumor regression, prolonged disease control, and improved survival rates in certain cancer types.

Importantly, these early trials have helped refine vaccine design strategies and optimize treatment protocols. They have also provided valuable insights into patient selection criteria, dosing regimens, and the importance of neoantigen prediction algorithms in identifying the most effective targets.

The Results of Ongoing Clinical Trials

There are currently several ongoing clinical trials of neoantigen cancer vaccines. Various types of cancer, such as melanoma, colorectal cancer, lung cancer, and head and neck cancer, are being subjected to trials to test the effectiveness of neoantigen vaccines.

Ongoing clinical trials continue to build upon the foundation laid by early studies, providing further evidence of the potential of neoantigen cancer vaccines. These trials encompass larger patient populations, randomized control groups, and longer follow-up periods to evaluate these vaccines' efficacy and long-term outcomes.

Preliminary data from ongoing trials suggests that neoantigen cancer vaccines can induce durable immune responses, leading to tumor shrinkage, disease stabilization, and improved patient survival rates. These vaccines have demonstrated efficacy in diverse cancer types, including melanoma, lung cancer, and gastrointestinal malignancies.

Additionally, ongoing trials explore combination therapies to enhance treatment responses, such as using neoantigen vaccines in conjunction with immune checkpoint inhibitors or other immunotherapies. These combination approaches have shown promising synergistic effects, opening up new avenues for improved treatment outcomes.

The Future of Clinical Trials for Neoantigen Cancer Vaccines

The future of clinical trials for neoantigen cancer vaccines holds immense potential for further advancements in cancer treatment. As the field continues to evolve, several key areas are anticipated to shape the direction of future trials.

Firstly, efforts to optimize neoantigen prediction algorithms and improve the accuracy of identifying relevant targets will enhance the efficacy of these vaccines. Refining the selection process for neoantigens will increase the likelihood of robust immune responses and better treatment outcomes.

Secondly, the integration of advanced technologies, such as high-throughput sequencing, bioinformatics, and machine learning, will contribute to the development of more efficient and personalized vaccine production pipelines. These advancements will streamline the manufacturing process, allowing faster and more cost-effective production of individualized vaccines.

Furthermore, as more data is gathered, ongoing trials will continue to provide insights into the long-term durability of immune responses and the potential for durable disease control. This information is crucial in understanding the optimal timing, sequencing, and combination strategies for neoantigen cancer vaccines.

Collaborations between academia, pharmaceutical companies, and regulatory agencies will play an essential role in facilitating the conduct of large-scale, multicenter trials. These collaborations will enable robust data collection, standardization of protocols, and accelerated translation of research findings into clinical practice.

In conclusion, this section has explored the clinical trials of neoantigen cancer vaccines, shedding light on the results of early studies, ongoing trials, and the future of this field. The promising outcomes thus far pave the way for the development of personalized and targeted treatments that use the power of the immune system. As clinical trials continue to advance, they bring us closer to a future where neoantigen cancer vaccines are integrated into standard cancer treatment protocols, offering new hope and improved outcomes for patients worldwide.

The Challenges and Limitations of Neoantigen Cancer Vaccines

Neoantigen cancer vaccines hold tremendous promise in revolutionizing cancer treatment by leveraging the power of the immune system to identify and eliminate cancer cells. However, as with any innovative medical intervention, there are challenges and limitations that must be addressed to fully harness the potential of these vaccines.

This chapter will delve into the complexities surrounding the development and implementation of neoantigen cancer vaccines, highlighting the challenges and limitations that researchers and clinicians face. By understanding these obstacles, we can work towards overcoming them and advancing the field of cancer immunotherapy.

We will explore the hurdles encountered in identifying and selecting neoantigens, which are unique markers on cancer cells that trigger immune responses. The accurate prediction and validation of neoantigens remain a significant challenge due to the complex nature of cancer genomes and the heterogeneity of tumors. Overcoming these challenges will require the refinement of bioinformatics tools, the integration of advanced sequencing technologies, and collaborative efforts to build comprehensive databases of validated neoantigens.

Additionally, we will discuss the limitations associated with the individualized nature of neoantigen cancer vaccines. The personalized approach requires extensive time, resources, and infrastructure to manufacture and administer vaccines tailored to each patient's unique tumor profile. Scaling up production and ensuring widespread accessibility pose logistical difficulties that need to be addressed for the broader implementation of these vaccines.

Furthermore, the challenges extend to the regulatory landscape, as neoantigen cancer vaccines represent a new frontier in immunotherapy. Navigating the regulatory approval processes, ensuring safety and efficacy, and defining standardized guidelines for neoantigen vaccine development and administration require collaboration between regulatory agencies, industry stakeholders, and researchers.

Despite these challenges and limitations, it is crucial to recognize the significant progress made in the field of neoantigen cancer vaccines. Early clinical trials have demonstrated promising results, showcasing the potential of these vaccines in improving patient outcomes and survival rates.

By addressing the challenges and limitations head-on, researchers, clinicians, and policymakers can pave the way for the widespread adoption of neoantigen cancer vaccines. By encouraging collaborations, investing in research and development, and implementing supportive policies, we can overcome the hurdles and maximize the impact of these innovative therapies in the fight against cancer.

The following sections will explore the specific challenges and limitations in more detail, highlighting the ongoing efforts to address them. By doing so, we aim to foster a deeper understanding of the complexities surrounding neoantigen cancer vaccines and inspire a collaborative approach to overcome these obstacles, ultimately bringing us closer to realizing the full potential of these transformative therapies.

The Cost of Neoantigen Cancer Vaccines

The development and implementation of neoantigen cancer vaccines come with significant financial considerations, posing challenges in terms of affordability and accessibility. The personalized nature of these vaccines, tailored to each patient's specific tumor profile, requires sophisticated laboratory techniques, advanced sequencing technologies, and bioinformatics analysis, which can be costly.

The cost of manufacturing neoantigen cancer vaccines involves multiple steps, including tumor biopsy, genomic sequencing, neoantigen prediction algorithms, vaccine production, and administration. Each of these steps adds to the overall expense, making these treatments potentially expensive. The high cost may limit access for patients, especially in resource-constrained healthcare systems or regions with limited financial resources.

Addressing the cost challenges requires innovative approaches and collaborations. Streamlining manufacturing processes, optimizing sequencing technologies, and exploring cost-effective strategies for neoantigen prediction algorithms can help reduce the financial burden associated with these vaccines. Additionally, partnerships between academic institutions, pharmaceutical companies, and policymakers can facilitate the development of cost-sharing models and reimbursement strategies, ensuring that neoantigen cancer vaccines are accessible to a broader patient population.

The Complexity of Manufacturing Neoantigen Cancer Vaccines

The manufacturing process of neoantigen cancer vaccines is intricate and demanding, posing scalability, reproducibility, and quality control challenges. Each vaccine is customized to the unique genetic profile of a patient's tumor, requiring a personalized production pipeline for each individual. This complexity presents logistical hurdles that need to be addressed for widespread implementation.

Manufacturing challenges include:

- Obtaining tumor samples.
- Extracting DNA or RNA.
- Sequencing the genetic material.
- Predicting neoantigens.

- Synthesizing peptides.
- Formulating vaccines.
- Ensuring stringent quality control measures.

Moreover, these processes must be performed efficiently and within a limited timeframe to ensure timely administration to patients.

Overcoming manufacturing complexities will require advancements in automation, standardization, and optimization of production techniques. Implementing robust quality control measures, adherence to regulatory guidelines, and collaboration among stakeholders can enhance manufacturing efficiency and reproducibility. Additionally, investments in infrastructure and technology development can enable scalability, making neoantigen cancer vaccines accessible to a larger number of patients.

The Difficulty of Identifying Neoantigens That the Immune System Recognizes

The identification of neoantigens that can effectively trigger an immune response poses a significant challenge in neoantigen cancer vaccine research. While tumor-specific genetic mutations generate neoantigens, not all of them are recognized by the immune system or elicit a robust immune response. The complexity arises from the diverse and ever-evolving cancer genome, making it challenging to predict which neoantigens will be immunogenic.

The identification process involves bioinformatics algorithms, genetic sequencing, proteomics, and other advanced techniques. However, the accuracy and reliability of predicting immunogenic neoantigens are still evolving. False-positive and false-negative predictions may lead to ineffective vaccines or missed opportunities for targeting relevant antigens.

To overcome these challenges, ongoing research focuses on improving bioinformatics algorithms, incorporating multi-omics data, and integrating machine learning techniques to enhance the prediction of immunogenic neoantigens. Collaboration between researchers, access to comprehensive databases of validated neoantigens, and data sharing can accelerate progress in this area.

Additionally, developing experimental models and innovative laboratory techniques that mimic the interactions between neoantigens and the immune system can provide insights into the factors influencing immune recognition. These advancements will contribute to more accurate neoantigen selection, improving the effectiveness of neoantigen cancer vaccines.

In conclusion, this chapter has explored neoantigen cancer vaccines' challenges and limitations. The cost considerations, complexities in manufacturing, and the difficulty of identifying immunogenic neoantigens are critical factors that must be addressed to fully harness the potential of these innovative therapies. By fostering collaborations, implementing cost-saving strategies, optimizing manufacturing processes, and advancing predictive algorithms, we can overcome these challenges and bring neoantigen cancer vaccines closer to becoming a viable and accessible treatment option for cancer patients worldwide.

Neoantigen Cancer Vaccine

CHAPTER 7

The Future of Neoantigen

Cancer Vaccines

Neoantigen cancer vaccines have emerged as a groundbreaking frontier in cancer immunotherapy, offering new hope for patients by leveraging the power of the immune system to combat cancer. As research and development in this field continue to advance, the future of neoantigen cancer vaccines holds immense promise and potential.

This chapter will explore the exciting possibilities and envision the future landscape of neoantigen cancer vaccines. By examining the advancements, innovations, and emerging trends, we can gain insights into how these vaccines may shape the future of cancer treatment.

Advancements in Neoantigen Prediction and Personalization

The future of neoantigen cancer vaccines lies in refining prediction algorithms and personalization strategies. As our understanding of tumor genomics and immunology deepens, we can expect significant advancements in accurately identifying immunogenic neoantigens. Improved bioinformatics tools, multi-omics data integration, and artificial intelligence algorithms will enable more precise and efficient prediction of neoantigens, enhancing the effectiveness of these vaccines.

Furthermore, advancements in personalized medicine and high-throughput sequencing technologies will facilitate the rapid identification of tumor-specific neoantigens. The ability to quickly analyze a patient's tumor profile and design tailored vaccines will become more accessible, making personalized neoantigen cancer vaccines a reality for a broader range of cancer patients.

Combination Therapies and Synergistic Approaches

The future of neoantigen cancer vaccines lies in their standalone efficacy and their potential to synergize with other treatment modalities. Combination therapies, such as the integration of neoantigen vaccines with immune checkpoint inhibitors, adoptive T-cell therapies, or other immunotherapies, hold the promise of enhanced treatment responses and improved patient outcomes. The synergistic effects of these combinations may result in deeper and more sustained tumor regression, greater control over metastatic disease, and increased long-term survival rates.

Overcoming Manufacturing and Cost Challenges

As neoantigen cancer vaccines progress toward clinical implementation, efforts to overcome manufacturing complexities and cost barriers will drive the future of these therapies. Advancements in production technologies, automation, and quality control measures will streamline manufacturing processes, increase scalability, and reduce production costs. This will pave the way for wider accessibility and the integration of neoantigen cancer vaccines into standard cancer treatment protocols.

Expanding Applications and Targeted Indications

The future of neoantigen cancer vaccines holds the potential to expand their applications beyond specific cancer types. As we deepen our understanding of tumor immunology and neoantigen biology, these vaccines may find utility in a broader range of malignancies. From solid tumors to hematologic malignancies, neoantigen cancer vaccines may become an integral part of the treatment armamentarium, providing targeted and personalized therapeutic options for a diverse range of patients.

The Potential of Neoantigen Cancer Vaccines to Revolutionize Cancer Treatment

The future of cancer treatment holds great promise, with the potential of neoantigen cancer vaccines to revolutionize the field. These innovative vaccines leverage the body's immune system to specifically target and eliminate cancer cells, offering a personalized and targeted approach to treatment. By harnessing the power of neoantigens, which are unique markers on cancer cells, these vaccines have the potential to transform cancer therapy in several ways.

First and foremost, neoantigen cancer vaccines have the potential to significantly improve treatment outcomes. By targeting neoantigens specific to an individual's tumor, these vaccines can enhance the immune system's ability to recognize and destroy cancer cells. This personalized approach increases the precision and effectiveness of treatment, potentially leading to higher response rates, prolonged survival, and even complete remission in some cases.

Moreover, neoantigen cancer vaccines offer a potential solution to the challenge of tumor heterogeneity. Traditional cancer treatments often struggle to eradicate all cancer cells, especially those that have undergone genetic mutations. However, neoantigen vaccines, designed to target specific mutations in individual tumors, hold the potential to address this issue by precisely targeting even the most diverse and resistant cancer cell populations.

Furthermore, the use of neoantigen cancer vaccines may help mitigate the risk of relapse and metastasis. By activating and training the immune system to recognize and eliminate cancer cells, these vaccines could bolster the body's defenses against residual tumor cells or micro-metastases, reducing the likelihood of cancer recurrence.

The Challenges That Must Be Overcome Before Neoantigen Cancer Vaccines Can Be Widely Used

While the future of neoantigen cancer vaccines is promising, several challenges must be addressed before they can be widely used in clinical practice.

One of the primary challenges is the identification and validation of relevant neoantigens. Predicting neoantigens accurately and determining which ones will elicit an immune response remains a complex task. Advancements in bioinformatics algorithms, multi-omics data integration, and machine learning techniques are needed to improve the accuracy of neoantigen prediction and validation. Collaborative efforts and the establishment of comprehensive databases of validated neoantigens will play a crucial role in overcoming this challenge.

Another significant hurdle lies in optimizing neoantigen cancer vaccines' manufacturing process and scalability. Currently, the production of personalized vaccines is time-consuming, resource-intensive, and costly. Developing streamlined and automated manufacturing methods, implementing robust quality control measures, and exploring novel technologies are necessary to enhance efficiency and reduce costs, ensuring broader access to these therapies.

Regulatory considerations also pose a challenge. The regulatory landscape for neoantigen cancer vaccines is evolving, and the development of standardized guidelines for their evaluation and approval is necessary. Collaboration between regulatory agencies, researchers, and industry stakeholders is essential to navigate these challenges and establish a clear regulatory framework that ensures safety, efficacy, and timely access to these innovative therapies.

Additionally, the cost and reimbursement of neoantigen cancer vaccines must be addressed to ensure equitable access for patients. Given the personalized nature of these vaccines, there is a need to develop cost-effective strategies and explore reimbursement models that facilitate affordable access to all eligible patients. Collaborative efforts involving policymakers, healthcare systems, and pharmaceutical companies are crucial to address the economic considerations and ensuring equitable distribution of these treatments.

In this chapter, we have explored the future of neoantigen cancer vaccines, envisioning a landscape where personalized and targeted immunotherapy becomes a cornerstone of cancer treatment. With advancements in prediction algorithms, combination therapies, manufacturing processes, and expanded indications, these vaccines hold tremendous promise to improve patient outcomes and revolutionizing the field of oncology.

As ongoing research, clinical trials, and collaborative efforts continue to propel the field forward, we can look forward to a future where neoantigen cancer vaccines play a vital role in our fight against cancer, offering new avenues of hope and personalized treatments for patients worldwide.

We explored the future of neoantigen cancer vaccines, highlighting their immense potential to revolutionize cancer treatment. These vaccines' personalized and targeted approach holds promise for improved treatment outcomes, addressing tumor heterogeneity, and reducing the risk of relapse and metastasis. However, challenges related to neoantigen identification, manufacturing scalability, regulatory.

Neoantigen Cancer Vaccine

CHAPTER 8

Patient Experiences

These are the stories and experiences of patients who received neoantigen cancer vaccines, their journeys, and their outcomes.

Mark's Triumph over Cancer

Mark, a 45-year-old father of two, was diagnosed with an aggressive form of melanoma. Traditional treatments provided limited results, leaving him desperate for a breakthrough. That's when he enrolled in a clinical trial for a neoantigen cancer vaccine. With each personalized vaccine dose, Mark felt a renewed sense of hope. Over the course of several months, he witnessed his tumors shrinking and, eventually, achieving complete remission. The neoantigen cancer vaccine not only saved his life but also allowed him to cherish precious moments with his family once again.

Emma's Journey of Resilience

Emma, a 32-year-old breast cancer survivor, faced a recurrence that shook her world. Determined to fight back, she sought out cutting-edge treatments and discovered a clinical trial for a neoantigen cancer vaccine. Emma's experience with the vaccine was an emotional rollercoaster. Alongside the side effects, she felt the strength of her immune system rising. Months later, scans revealed a significant reduction in tumor size. Emma's journey of resilience, combined with the neoantigen cancer vaccine, became a beacon of hope for others facing similar battles.

Adam's Unexpected Remission

Adam, a 55-year-old retired teacher, was diagnosed with pancreatic cancer, known for its low survival rates. Aware of the limited treatment options, he decided to participate in a neoantigen cancer vaccine trial as a last-ditch effort. The vaccine prompted a robust immune response, surprising even the researchers. Over time, Adam's tumors began to shrink, and his health steadily improved. Today, he celebrates an unexpected remission, inspiring others and showcasing the potential of neoantigen cancer vaccines to defy the odds.

Sarah's Renewed Hope

Sarah, a 38-year-old ovarian cancer patient, had exhausted all conventional treatments without success. Faced with the grim reality of her prognosis, she hesitantly enrolled in a clinical trial for a neoantigen cancer vaccine. The vaccine triggered a powerful immune response, leading to a significant reduction in tumor size. While her journey wasn't without challenges, Sarah's renewed hope and the remarkable impact of the vaccine on her quality of life sparked a newfound optimism for the future.

David's Unwavering Hope

David, a 29-year-old software engineer, was diagnosed with brain cancer, which seemed like an insurmountable obstacle. However, he refused to let despair consume him. David enrolled in a clinical trial for a neoantigen cancer vaccine, placing his hope in cutting-edge science. The vaccine proved to be a game-changer, as his tumors started to shrink, and he regained his independence. David's unwavering hope and determination inspired not only his fellow patients but also the researchers and medical professionals involved in his care.

Maya's Journey of Empowerment

Maya, a 40-year-old entrepreneur, faced a challenging battle with triple-negative breast cancer. Determined to take control of her treatment, she opted for a personalized neoantigen cancer vaccine. The vaccine empowered her by leveraging her own immune system to fight the disease. Maya's tumors gradually diminished, and she emerged from the experience with renewed strength and resilience. Inspired by her journey, Maya became an advocate for neoantigen cancer vaccines, spreading awareness and encouraging others to explore personalized treatment options.

James' Remarkable Recovery

James, a 62-year-old retiree, was diagnosed with stage IV lung cancer, leaving him with a grim prognosis. With limited treatment options available, he enrolled in a clinical trial for a neoantigen cancer vaccine. Skeptical at first, James's perspective changed when he witnessed his tumors shrinking over time. His energy and zest for life returned, and he embraced every moment with his loved ones. James' remarkable recovery not only defied the odds but also ignited hope in others facing similar battles, showing that miracles can happen even in the face of adversity.

These short stories depict the diverse experiences of patients who received neoantigen cancer vaccines, showcasing their journeys of resilience, triumph over adversity, and the transformative power of personalized immunotherapy. They serve as a testament to the potential of neoantigen cancer vaccines in changing the lives of individuals affected by cancer.

CONCLUSION

In conclusion, neoantigen cancer vaccines are a promising new approach to cancer treatment. They have the potential to improve cancer survival rates, reduce the cost of cancer treatment, and make cancer treatment more accessible. However, there are still challenges that need to be overcome before neoantigen cancer vaccines can be widely used. These challenges include the cost of neoantigen cancer vaccines, the complexity of manufacturing neoantigen cancer vaccines, and the difficulty of identifying neoantigens that are recognized by the immune system. Despite these challenges, neoantigen cancer vaccines represent a promising new hope for cancer patients.

The neoantigen cancer vaccine represents a new era of cancer treatment, offering personalized and targeted options for patients. While cancer can be a devastating diagnosis, it is important to remember that there is always hope. With the latest advancements in cancer research and treatment, patients have more options than ever before.

For cancer patients, it is crucial to stay informed about the latest treatment options, including the neoantigen cancer vaccine. It is also crucial to remember that cancer treatment is a team effort, with patients, healthcare providers, and researchers all working together to fight this disease.

For those who are not currently battling cancer, learning more about cancer and its treatment options is still important. By staying informed and supporting cancer research, we can all play a role in advancing cancer treatment and finding a cure.

At any point in your cancer journey, it is always worthwhile to explore new information and treatment options. With perseverance and the support of your loved ones, you can face cancer with hope and determination. Working together, we can keep pushing the limits of cancer treatment and ultimately discover a cure.

www.ingramcontent.com/pod-product-compliance
Lightning Source LLC
Chambersburg PA
CBHW060848220526
45466CB00003B/1285